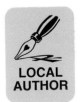

STRUCTURED SPINNING *for* SENIORS

AND THOSE WHO WANT TO BE SENIORS

Joel J. Malek

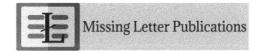

Missing Letter Publications

Published by:

Missing Letter Publications

PORT WASHINGTON, NEW YORK

ISBNs: 979-8-9852469-0-2 (softcover)
979-8-9852469-1-9 (ebook)

Typesetting and cover design: Gary A. Rosenberg

Printed in the United States of America

This guide is dedicated to our healthcare workers,
all of whom sacrificed and suffered through the
past year and months of the COVID-19 pandemic,
and especially to those workers who gave all.

And to my wife, Patricia, who motivated and inspired me
throughout my book-writing journey with her spin-related
comments and her own rigor in the gym.

Contents

CHAPTER 1

Welcome to Structured Spinning

The intention of this guide is to introduce "seniors" to the physical activity commonly known today as spinning and to present my own spinning methodology: Structured Spinning. Besides the methodology, included within this guide are the basic equipment needs, spinning moves, workout structure, and so on. For a quick look at the contents of each chapter, read the chapter summary.

So why spinning? Somewhere around 1998 and at the age of forty-seven, after decades of skiing and playing competitive racquetball, my knees began to signal me that I'd soon be hanging up my racquet and finding some other use for those little blue balls I'd been splitting over the years. A visit to the orthopedist confirmed a tear in my left medial meniscus and arthritis in my right knee, so something was going to have to change in the not-too-distant future. Also, around this time I began to notice the spinning studio classes at the racquet club and also what appeared to be a steady increase in class size. I had always enjoyed outdoor cycling and wondered about this "new" type of indoor cycling exercise and whether it could deliver the same level of cardio workout I was used to on the racquetball court and possibly help my ailing knees.

About a year passed and my orthopedist advised that it was time to get off the racquetball court and look for something else. And, as you might have guessed, he recommended indoor cycling as a good therapy for my knees. I gave it a try, and soon I was a regular in the spinning classes. My knees began to feel better, and I could tell that the cardio workout I was looking for was in reach if I continued to attend the 45-minute-long classes twice and then three times a week. I also realized other benefits that supported my longevity on the ski slopes, and these continue today without any surgery, cortisone shots, or other medical intervention.

So, what is this panacea? Spinning—and what is Structured Spinning, where does it come from, and why is it something that seniors, and those wanting to be seniors, should consider? First, spinning is an indoor cycling exercise that mimics outdoor road cycling like that seen in the famous Tour de France. That is not to say that you will be training for such an arduous feat as the Tour de France, but I use the Tour just to give you a general idea of what the activity of spinning is like as opposed to using an indoor gym bicycle, the latter of which does not support pedaling while out of the saddle/seat (i.e., standing rather than sitting while turning the bike peddles). An indoor gym bicycle is designed more for still or stationary peddling while in a seated position. In contrast, spinning cycles are designed for both in-the-saddle and out-of-the saddle positions, and also for a more rigorous workout as one might imagine while mimicking cycling through the Green Mountains of Vermont or in the French Pyrenees as with the Tour de France. This distinction between stationary gym bicycling and spinning will become more important as I discuss equipment and workouts in later chapters.

Second, I define Structured Spinning as a method that I developed and use to ensure that I'm achieving the highest maximum workout from my spin session on any given day. It is a method of pushing oneself by measuring key factors like heart rate, while staying within individual health guidelines based on age, condition, energy level, and spin training, on any given day. It is a commonsense approach that recognizes that, on any given day, any one of us may not be up to a loud head-banging 60-minute high-intensity class, but instead be more comfortable spinning twice for 15 minutes and at a lower intensity level.

Structured Spinning is also a method of insuring consistency from one spin session workout to the next. But regardless of what kind of spin workout you do or need today, you must understand what you are able to accomplish each time you spin in order to maintain and improve the level of your spin workout over time. Structured Spinning accomplishes this by utilizing several components to measure and gauge performance throughout a session. The three basic measurement essentials are heart rate, time, and spin cycle revolutions per minute (RPMs) or "cadence." In addition, Structured Spinning also recognizes such ride components as saddle position, moves, and incline/resistance, and their impact on the three basic measurement essentials.

You may be wondering about spin classes and why not just attend these? The short answer is that after attending classes religiously for the first five years, I realized that they generally do not follow much structure, particularly regarding consistency from session to session. You rarely have the same instructor from day to day, so there's little consistency between sessions, and there may or may not be any consideration of heart rate, cadence/RPMs, etc., by the instructor du jour. Besides not satisfying these basic needs, for me, the classes eventually became a scheduling inconvenience, very annoying, and in several ways unhealthy.

Yes, unhealthy, which is pretty mind-blowing since most of the time spinning classes are attended at a *health* club! First, it's rare to find a class where the music is played at a healthy decibel level. Countless times, I would leave class and complain to the management about the head-splitting volume levels at which music was being played. I'd ask how they could justify playing the music at such an unhealthy decibel level at a health club. They'd just shrug their shoulders and give some nonsensical answer, totally ignoring the inconsistency. It didn't end there.

Another "unhealthy" practice I've encountered at many studios and complained to management about is the practice of spinning in a dark studio. How bizarre: One club's spin studio had glow-in-the-dark paint under a black light. I felt like I was in a disco on Friday night rather than a spin studio to get a workout. In the dark studio, it is often impossible to read heart rate monitors, the cadence displayed, incline/resistance, seat-height settings, etc. I'd ask to have the lights turned on so that I could read my heart rate monitor, the RPM, watts, and time display on the bike.

But, usually, my request would fall on deaf ears because the instructor found it more important to create some kind of hocus-pocus transcendental mood or a simulated "night ride" or booming disco or who knows what. Ridiculous.

So, over time, I found spin class to be both disappointing and annoying: instructors yelling out orders like drill sergeants with such cliches as "Make it burn!" or "Go for it!" and my favorite, "Make it your ride!" Come on now—in spin class, it's never MY ride; it's the instructor's! The instructor controls everything—the moves, the cadence, the music and lights, and the duration, stretching (often overlooked and skipped), all the while ignoring the important stuff like targeted cadence, incline/resistance level, and where your heart rate should be for a given period of time. In reality, it was the instructor's ride, and we were just "along for the ride." But now I'm going to show you that it doesn't have to be this way because with Structured Spinning, I'll teach you how to really make it *your* ride.

If this sounds like something for you, I'm betting that eventually the day will come, as it did with me, that you will want to spin but can't make class; or maybe you're just tired of being yelled at over ear-blistering music, or perhaps you're new to spinning and would like to avoid classes all together. In my case, when the day came that I couldn't make the scheduled class, I decided to just get on a bike by myself, plug in my headphones, and start doing my own ride. I had done plenty of class sessions and knew all the moves. Before I knew it, it was just like what they always said in class . . . I finally made it MY ride. I didn't need to be in a class to do a spin session, and soon I began to realize how much more I enjoyed my own sessions.

A little while later, I began to realize how the different components of spinning—i.e., time/duration, heart rate, incline/resistance, and cadence RPMs—give structure to a spin session and how they are related to the different spin moves. Not unlike athletic training, this structure provided a self-motivating platform principled in repeatable, consistent, measurable, improved performance, and planned workout sessions. You learn to maintain and achieve new levels using the key element of heart rate, duration, incline/resistance, and cadence. This is what Structured Spinning is about, and what follows in this guide is how you can adopt it, make it your own, and spin without ever having to endure another dark, deafening, senseless, and often disappointing spin class.

Since one of the guiding principles of Structured Spinning is to truly make it your ride, it is easily adapted to any age, making it an excellent exercise for seniors and those approaching their senior years. It is a great **low-impact cardiovascular workout**, and as I mentioned earlier, I began spinning at the age of forty-seven and continue spinning today as I turn seventy. But, if you are above age forty, I strongly encourage you to talk with your doctor or even ask your doctor to read through this guide and get their OK before you give it a go. I know plenty of people with many more years than I who include spinning regularly in their workouts as I do. Despite this, again, I caution you to discuss spinning with your physician.

Finally, the reason seniors and those wanting to become seniors should consider Structured Spinning is that there are too many health benefits to ignore for both men and women in the age band I mentioned. As we've played and enjoyed life over the years, our knees, heart, muscle groups, shape, and size have aged and will continue to age whether or not we notice it. Not only does spinning benefit your muscles— everything from your legs to your core—but as I've said it's also a great low-impact cardiovascular workout, which improves your blood flow, increases your stamina, boosts your mood, and reduces the likelihood you will suffer from chronic issues such as high blood pressure, heart disease, stroke, and diabetes.

Spinning uses all the major lower-body muscles—the glutes, hamstrings, quads, shins, and calves. A study by the American Council On Exercise found that, during spinning, individuals worked at 75–96% of their maximum heart rate[1]—far exceeding the minimum requirement. The fixed wheel of a spin bike means you can't "freewheel," so your muscles work the whole time. This makes it a pretty high-intensity

---

1 AceFitness.Org. "Indoor Cycling, America's Hottest Fitness Craze, Geared for the Conditioned, New ACE Study Finds," October 19, 1997, https://www.acefitness.org/about-ace/press-room/press-releases/225/indoor-cycling-america-s-hottest-fitness-craze-geared-for-the-conditioned-new-ace-study-finds/, accessed September 13, 2021.

activity that burns a lot of calories. The health benefits are real and very much in reach for many seniors, simply because of the low-impact nature of the spinning workout.

I'm going to show you how to ease into it, so don't be intimidated or turned off by what you've seen/heard coming from your club's spin studio. If you can ride a bicycle, it's likely, with an OK from your doctor, that you are ready to try spinning on your own or in a health club spin class. Health club classes are a good place to start, but I encourage you to get a jump start by reading this guide before you go. You'll learn about the equipment, setting up the bike, and the basic spin positions and moves in Chapter 3. If you don't like what you see and hear in the health club spin studio, keep reading, and I'll show you how to spin on your own. From the start, you can have it your way, versus the one-size-fits-all approach in a spin class. So, take a "just do it" approach and get ready to move and move out of the noise and into the Structured Spinning groove, at home, in the gym, and/or while traveling.

CHAPTER 1 SUMMARY

The author explains why he "migrated" to spinning more than twenty years ago and the roots of the Structured Spinning methodology, its health benefits, and its guiding principles.

CHAPTER 2

Starting Out: Equipment

Before you do anything, you *must* make sure that your doctor approves of your decision to give spinning a try. Spinning can be an aggressive physical workout that will challenge both the cardiorespiratory and musculoskeletal systems of the body. Besides demanding more from your heart and lungs, spinning will stress the body's bones (the skeleton), muscles, cartilage, tendons, ligaments, joints, and other connective tissue that supports and binds tissues and organs together. I cannot emphasize enough the need to be safe and check with your physician before starting, regardless of your age and physical condition. Once you've been given the OK by your physician, you'll need some knowledge of spinning equipment to get started. Here's a look at what you'll need.

EQUIPMENT

The basic equipment used for spinning includes workout clothes, spin shoes or sneakers, spin bike, and various monitoring gear (to measure time, heart rate, RPM/cadence, incline/resistance, etc.). Keep in mind that, in any sport or activity, the equipment will evolve and change as design/manufacturing improvements are made, consumer tastes change, technology develops, and so on. So, some online and/or periodical research of the latest trends in spinning (e.g., *Cycling Weekly*) is warranted before you spend your money. However, if you are a beginner and planning to try spinning at your health club, all you really need to start a spinning program are sneakers and whatever you're comfortable wearing in the gym. This will get you started; however, to pursue Structured Spinning, you will need to consider the equipment addressed below.

If you are, however, someone who already spins and you want to learn about Structured Spinning, jump ahead to Chapter 4.

To follow the Structured Spinning methodology, you will need to have three basic pieces of equipment. Two are essential: 1) a spin bike and 2) a heart rate monitor (or other means of monitoring your heart rate during the spin session). The third, spinning shoes, will become important to wear as your session time and intensity increase. Once you are spinning three or more days a week for more than 30 to 40 minutes a session, sneakers will become uncomfortable, and you'll want the support of spinning shoes (aka cycling shoes). The support they provide will enable more rigorous and longer sessions without aching feet.

Spin Shoes

I've been using spin shoes made by Specialized for many years. In fact, they are the only brand I've ever used. I find they are reasonably priced (under $100), durable, long lasting, and fit me well. You can pay a lot more or a little less, but, in any case, you should do some research and try a few in a cycle shop before you buy. Of similar quality and price are Nike and Shimano, and you'll find a wide selection with year 2021 reviews by visiting www.bestreviews.guide. Also, the cleats on the bottom of a cycling shoe are what enables you, the rider, to connect the spin shoe on your foot to the bike peddle (aka to clip in). Initially, you will have to buy a pair of cleats. They are usually an additional charge ($10, more or less), but they are reusable, so if you have a pair of old spin shoes, you can remove the cleats using an Allen key and screw them on to your new shoes. I've only owned one pair of cleats in my spinning lifetime.

Heart Rate Monitors & Spin Bikes

That's all I'll say about spinning shoes, so let's look at the two essential pieces of equipment to Structured Spinning: a heart rate monitoring device and spin bike. If you are lucky to find or own a spin bike that includes an onboard heart rate monitoring device, you are all set. Most of the time, however, you'll need or want for convenience your own heart rate monitoring device. As I mentioned in Chapter 1, Structured Spinning is principled in three key measurements: heart rate, cadence, and time. Ideally then, a spin bike will incorporate a device or devices that will provide or support these three measurements. Unfortunately, most or many spin bikes support none or only one or two; however, the problem can be solved by locating a clock on the studio wall or on your phone, etc., and owning your own heart rate monitor. I'll return later to discuss cadence/RPM.

What I mean when I say that some spin bikes support heart rate monitoring is that some spin bikes can support the wireless transmittal of your heart rate from a personal heart rate monitor to the bike display, when you are wearing a capable heart rate monitoring device during the session—e.g., the eSpinner bike by Star Trac, whose display is pictured below. This type of spin bike will support the monitoring of your heart rate if you are wearing a compatible heart rate transmitter. Also notice the enhanced graphics, time remaining, calories (burned), cadence (RPM), and other measures included on the eSpinner display.

Heart Rate Monitoring

Presently there are very few spin bikes that provide a full capability of reading your heart rate from the handlebar grip sensors and displaying it on its monitor—e.g., the Exerpeutic LX7. Or frequently now, some spin bikes come with their own transmitter strap, which connects to the bike's display; however, if you expect to spin while traveling, it's unlikely that this transmitter strap will work with another bike. More than likely, you'll have to compensate for the heart rate monitoring shortcoming of the bike you are using by owning and wearing your own heart rate monitoring device—e.g., wearing a $60 Polar FT1 will go a long way in being ready

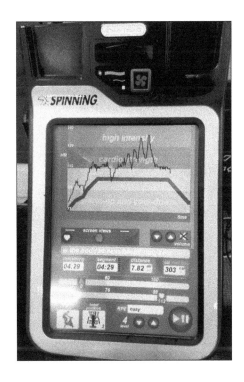

to execute a Structured Spin session anywhere regardless of the extent to which the spin bike provides or supports heart rate monitoring, and it will be useful in the gym weight room and during outside activities in observing your heart rate.

I've been using a MyZone MZ-3 Heart Rate Monitor (a physical activity chest belt with Bluetooth) for about a year and a half at the time of this writing. It "pairs" to its own app on my iPhone, as well as with the large MyZone wall display in the spin studio, and those on the gym walls making it easy to see and gauge the intensity of my workout outside the spin studio as well as while I'm spinning. There are several displays in the app. The basic includes actual heart rate as beats per minute (BPM), percentage to maximum heart rate, calorie burn, and other related graphics and info. You'll find this device priced around $100 plus or minus, if you shop around online. Check out all the MyZone products and features on their website.

Spin Bikes

Moving on from the heart rate monitoring discussion, it's important to realize that while heart rate monitoring is essential to Structured Spinning, there are other important features to consider with regard to the spin bike as the most important essential piece of equipment related to Structured Spinning. A good way to gauge how robust a spin bike is, is to compare the features you'll find on basic cycles and those with more robust capabilities. After you've solved the heart rate monitoring capability/shortcomings of a bike, moving up the capabilities ladder presented here will guide you toward the best bike available to you. To facilitate this discussion, I'm going to group spinning bikes into three categories: No Frills, Basic Display Capable, and Virtual Attendant.

No Frills–Surprisingly, many fitness/health clubs have bikes that don't include a display console, and therefore there is no onboard heart rate monitoring capability, no clock/time (remaining/elapsed), cadence/RPM, or incline/resistance level displays. This is not to say you can't support Structured Spinning on this kind of bike, you just need to adapt. I spend four months in Florida every winter, and the fitness club I use has a studio filled with Star Trac Spinner NXT bikes like the one pictured on the facing page.

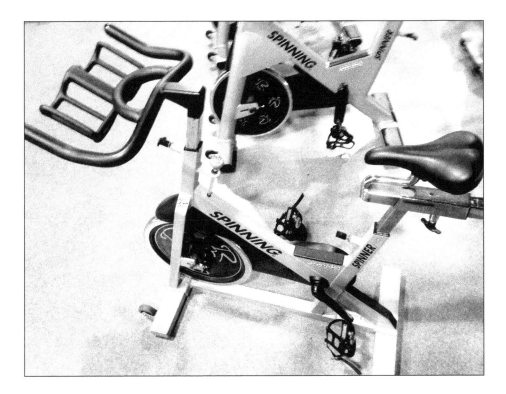

Star Trac Spinner NXT bike

Until recently, I used the clock on the wall for time durations, a Garmin Approach for heart rate monitoring; and I manually counted cadence/RPMs (more on cadence/counting below) and used the basic incline/resistance dial on the frame of the bike to judge perceived incline (more on perceived incline in Chapter 3).

Basic Display Capable—At the next level, a number of spin bikes have displays that include heart rate, cadence/RPM, incline/resistance, time elapsed, calories burned, watts, and distance. This level of spin bike does a good job of supporting Structured Spinning; however, you'll still need to have your own compatible heart rate transmitter, like that which comes with the Polar FT1 and others. Spin bikes like the eSpinner by Star Trac or the Keiser (pictured on the following page) will most likely pair with and read your transmitter if you are wearing one; but, otherwise, the bike, like most, is not equipped with handlebar or other such sensors.

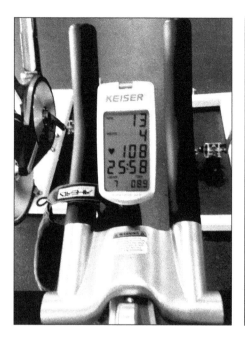 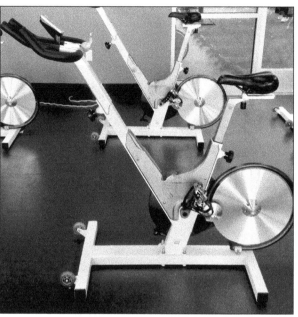

In any case, I'm not a fan of bikes that include heart rate sensors on the handlebar because these require that your hand position be kept constant. Once you move your hands, contact is lost and you'll lose the reading. A body-wearable transmitter and strap is the way to go here.

The basic display bikes I've mentioned will also support incline/resistance settings. However, some do not, in which case the incline/resistance level may be a "perceived" evaluation—i.e., it's something you, the rider, estimate based on the level of difficulty moving the bike peddles. This is commonly referred to as perceived exertion or perceived effort. But don't worry, I'll discuss how to gauge this in terms of "road incline," as if you were riding outdoors.

Virtual Attendant—In the high-end market of spin bikes, manufacturers like Peloton, Echelon, NordicTrack, Bowflex, and others, have introduced internet-connected bikes. Most require a monthly online class subscription in addition to the initial cost of the bike. Bikes at this level are primarily, possibly exclusively, for in-home use—i.e., it's very unlikely you will find any of these bikes in a health club spin studio, if for no other reason than they possibly compete with health clubs that offer spin classes as a reason to join the club.

The Virtual Attendant, or "connected" spin bikes, include an internet-connected display that places the rider virtually in the bike manufacturer's (or another subscription provider's) live scheduled spin class and/or gives them access to a catalog of online prerecorded classes. However, beyond the connectivity feature, the workout display features on these are reminiscent of the eSpinner bike by Star Trac shown above. For example, the Peloton bike utilizes a 20-inch-plus size display, which, besides seeing and hearing the spin instructor in virtual spin class, includes and improves on such measures as cadence and output watts by displaying current, average, and "best" reading for each stat. Also displayed is speed, distance, total output, calories, and incline/resistance. If the rider is wearing a compatible heart rate transmitter, heart rate is also displayed. In the end, the primary advancement here is the connection to a virtual class.

Other advances in this class of spin bike includes, from both the MYX Fitness and the no-subscription required Bowflex, a heart rate reading capability via an included rechargeable forearm monitor, and the NordicTrack S15i using a mechanical shaft to simulate the inclines and declines of actual bike riding.

Other spin bike amenities include programmed routine workouts, where the bike's software generates and changes incline/resistance levels during the ride session (eSpinner bike by Star Trac); handlebar and seat adjustment, leveling feet, and onboard cooling fans.

A final word about spin bikes

Should you decide to purchase one, take a good amount of time to read the reviews, try before you buy, and get a thirty-day return policy. I've heard from several who were disappointed in the quality and performance of their purchase, which resulted in a loss of interest (and money).

Apparel

Besides spin shoes and/or sneakers, the apparel you typically wear to the gym or to an exercise activity like Zumba, yoga, etc., will be fine for spinning. But be prepared to sweat, so lighter shorts and T-shirts, in addition to ancillaries such as a towel, water bottle, and head and/or wrist bands are recommended. For those suffering from arthritic-like joint ailments, do not hesitate to wear wrist supports, knee supports, and other supportive gear while spinning.

CHAPTER 2 SUMMARY

In this chapter, the author discusses why he considers spinning to be an aggressive physical workout, which challenges both the cardiorespiratory and musculoskeletal systems, and, therefore, for the beginner, it is a *must* to make sure that your doctor approves of your decision to give spinning a try. The remainder of the chapter examines equipment and apparel for Structured Spinning, including various heart rate monitors, spin shoes, bikes, apparel, and more.

CHAPTER 3

Spinning Basics

In the preceding two chapters you read about spinning as a cardiovascular exercise, got an overview of the principles of Structured Spinning methodology at the 30,000-foot level, and learned about the equipment involved and how it correlates to the Structured Spinning methodology. In this chapter, you'll learn what to check before getting on a spin bike and what's involved with setting it up, the basic spin positions, the moves and segments that make up a spin session, and two additional key elements of the spinning exercise: incline/resistance and cadence.

Along with time and duration, incline/resistance and cadence are what drive your heart rate and how hard you are working toward your workout goals—i.e., incline/resistance and cadence contribute in a big way toward optimizing and making it YOUR ride!

Cadence is the rate at which you are turning the bike pedals and its flywheel while incline/resistance is the level or degree of difficulty at which the pedals/flywheel are turned. The latter can be and is often associated with the incline that you'd experience bicycling outdoors in places like the Green Mountains of Vermont or competing in the Tour de France. The spin bike you have may or may not provide a way to monitor these two elements, so we'll look at ways to gauge these without the benefit of technology before I continue with spinning basics.

INCLINE/RESISTANCE

Incline/resistance is typically generated by applying resistance to the flywheel of the spin bike, which the bike accomplishes by using such means as an automotive-like brake pad, a tension belt around the flywheel, or more often today, by applying a magnetic force to the metallic flywheel. Typically, the rider changes the degree of incline/resistance by turning a small knob located near the handlebars, as seen on the Star Trac Spinner NXT photo, or by moving a lever forward and back to increase or decrease the incline/resistance, as seen on the Keiser photo in Chapter 2. These control mechanisms are easy to locate and use, and often the level of incline/resistance is displayed. However, on occasion, you'll come across a bike where there isn't any means to measure or gauge how much incline/resistance is being applied. On such bikes, the degree of incline/resistance is left to the rider's judgment—i.e., a perceived measurement—in which case the rider must judge incline/resistance by how the legs feel as more and less incline/resistance is applied through the moves and segments of the spin session. While these bikes are becoming rare, used over a short time, the rider will improve his/her perception and overcome this shortcoming of the bike.

So, in consideration of its importance to Structured Spinning, take the time to find a health club where the bikes will support the means of gauging and displaying a measure of incline/resistance. Having this capability will add an important degree of consistency to your workouts by enabling you to control the degree of difficulty through different moves and segments of a ride and to gauge your strength building and progress over time.

Today's spin bikes offer different measures to gauge incline/resistance—e.g., some gauge resistance in terms of recognized perceived exertion (RPE) as easy, moderate, or difficult; some bikes attempt to parallel road bikes using a degree of incline measure, or simply as a degree of difficulty 1 to 10. Bikes offering such measures of incline/resistance provide both a mechanism such as a knob or handle to apply the incline/resistance and a display that indicates the degree to which incline/resistance is being applied. Whatever you end up with, become familiar and comfortable with applying and controlling incline/resistance levels through YOUR ride.

CADENCE

As I mentioned earlier, cadence is the rate at which you turn the peddles/flywheel. Together with the incline/resistance applied to the flywheel, the rider can control the degree of difficulty of the ride and, consequently, heart rate. Many spin bikes measure and display cadence in terms of peddle/flywheel revolutions per minute (RPM). However, like incline/resistance, some bikes do not provide this measurement. But unlike the measure of incline/resistance, cadence can more easily be accurately gauged by the rider. This is done simply by counting revolutions as you turn the bike peddles, counting a single revolution, or stroke, as your left or right foot reaches the lowest point in the revolution. Using whatever you are using to measure time, count the number of times your foot reaches the low point of the stroke over a 15-second duration. If you are turning the peddles slowly and count just 10 revolutions during the 15 seconds, your revolutions per minute, RPM, is equal to 40 (10 revolutions times 4 equals 40 revolutions per minute), since there are four 15-second intervals in a minute. Once you've got this method of determining cadence, you will want to work at reaching and holding a cadence of 80 RPM, which is 20 strokes in 15 seconds. You can and should check your cadence throughout your spin session at any time by simply repeating a count of strokes for a 15-second period.

As with measuring incline/resistance, it's important to take the time to find a health club where the bikes support the measure and display of cadence. Having an easy means to gauge cadence through the spin session will increase consistency in your workouts by enabling you to control the degree of difficulty through different moves and segments of a ride and to gauge your strength building and progress over time.

So, now, before we discuss components like ride positions, moves, and segments, let's first check the bike and see that it's ready to ride.

BEFORE GETTING ON THE BIKE

Assuming that you've received medical clearance from your doctor; that you understand the features the bike has or doesn't have to support your measurement of time, cadence, incline/resistance, and heart rate; and that you are now dressed in appropriate workout clothes and footwear and ready to mount the bike and ride, we'll take a look at readying the bike itself.

This is also a good time to make sure you have a good supply of water at hand to keep yourself well hydrated through the ride and that you have a small hand towel to wipe away the sweat from your face. Most bikes will have a bottle rest for your water; the towel can be draped from the handlebars. Some riders find it comfortable to wear sweatbands on the forehead and/or wrists and joint supports.

Now let's inspect and set up the bike. You should not spin on a bike that is unlevel, "rocking," unstable, or broken in any way. It is both unsafe and uncomfortable, so check for broken components like a nonfunctioning incline/resistance knob, peddle foot straps, etc., as we go through the following bike setup.

Leveling the Bike

Placing one hand on the bike seat and the other on the handlebars, forcibly try to rock the bike back and forth, and side to side, to determine whether the bike is level. Again, you should not spin on a bike that is not level, "rocking," unstable, or broken in any way. If you find that the bike is not level, either move to another bike, assuming there are others in the spin studio, or adjust the leveling screw pads (i.e., the feet) at the bottom of the bike where it meets the floor. The bike may be too heavy for you to do this by yourself, but I often do it by getting a shoulder into the saddle or handlebars and tilt/lift it just enough to turn the leveling screws to correct the height. Typically, just a small turn will do the trick or sometimes a folded paper towel will do the trick. If this is not possible, find another bike or ask the club staff for assistance.

Seat Adjustment

All spin bikes have a means to adjust the seat up/down and forward/back. Proper seat adjustment is critical to a comfortable, safe, and efficient ride. If the seat height is too high, you will not be able to comfortably extend your leg properly during the power stroke. This can also lead to discomfort in the knees and hips. If the seat is too low, you will feel cramped and not be able to fully extend your legs, resulting in too much pressure on your knees and you won't be able to fully extend and utilize the strength of your quadriceps. Your seat should be adjusted such that when your foot reaches the bottom of the stroke, the knee-leg should be about 92 to 95% extended as illustrated in the picture at right.

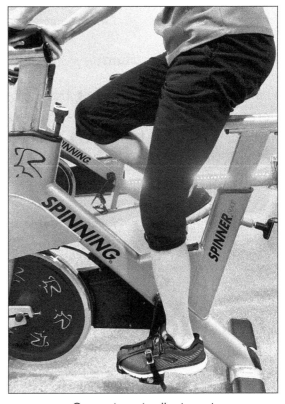

Correct seat adjustment

For starters, loosen the seat adjustment knob and move the seat up or down so that the top of the seat is at a height equal to the top of your hipbone while standing on the floor next to the seat. Set the height and get into the saddle. Clip in your spin shoes or place your sneakered feet into the peddle webbing (aka the basket). Turn the peddles and note your leg extension before making further adjustments to the seat height. You may have to get on and off a few times before you get the seat height right.

Now fine-tune your seat position by adjusting its forward/back setting; the adjustment knob will usually be found directly under and to the rear of the seat support frame. Take some time to make these critical adjustments, and again note the settings on the bike's frame where seat height, forward/back are indicated. Using a note app on your smartphone is a handy way to record these settings for the next time you spin.

Handlebars/Adjustment

Handlebars vary between bikes, but most often, a spin bike's handlebars will support two or three hand positions. I'll refer to these positions as: normal/flat, out, and extended. Take another look at the Keiser bike photo in Chapter 2. The first position, or normal/flat, is that area on the handlebar directly to the sides of the middle red incline/resistance lever; the out position is the handlebar area directly forward of the red incline/resistance lever, and the extended position is the point on the handlebar furthest forward and to the side of the red incline/resistance lever. Similar positioning is possible on virtually all spin bikes. We'll cover how these positions are used later. For now, let's continue setting up the bike by adjusting the height and extension of the handlebar to your seated "base" position.

All handlebars are easily adjusted for height. In some cases, like the Keiser bike pictured in Chapter 2, the adjustment will also result in changing the forward-back position of the handlebar—i.e., the space between the handlebar and the rider. All handlebars have a locking knob or other device that will unlock the position of the handlebar and allow the rider to move the handlebar up/down/out/in. Often, you will have to unscrew and pull the locking pin from its hole in the frame after loosening it to move the handlebar position. A number (or letter) setting on the frame will typically be found to mark the position, which you will be wise to remember or note down once you've found a comfortable setting.

For starters, move the handlebars to a position where you can easily reach out parallel to the floor and place your hands comfortably grabbing the handlebar while in the saddle. You'll likely have to adjust this a couple of times after mounting the bike and sitting in the saddle, until you find the setting that you are comfortable with over the duration of your ride. Once you've set these positions, make sure to tighten their screw-in pins.

Incline/Resistance Control Device

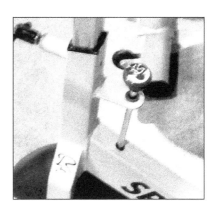

Finally, make sure you've located the incline/resistance control device, which is typically a knob or lever located adjacent to the handlebar. This knob (Star Trac Spinner NXT) or lever (Keiser bike) often indicates which direction will increase or decrease incline/resistance as in the picture at right.

MOUNTING THE BIKE, ENGAGING YOUR FEET TO THE PEDDLES, AND START SPINNING

If you're not sitting on the bike at this time, you'll want to mount the bike as you would any bicycle, make final adjustments as discussed above, and get yourself comfortably seated in the saddle. If this is your first time, be careful as the peddles will spin on their spindles, offering a "basket" for your sneakers to be slipped into,

or on the reverse bottom side, cleats for clipping in your spin shoes. You may have to rotate the peddle with the tip of your foot to get the peddle aligned to whichever kind of footwear you are wearing. Your feet *must* be "attached" to the peddles, using either the peddle baskets or by clipping your spin shoes into the cleats as seen in the photo on the next page.

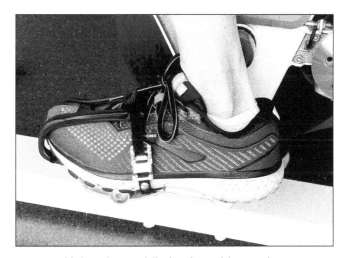

Using the peddle basket with sneaker

Now set the incline/resistance so that it will be easy (7+/– of 30) to turn the peddles and place your hands on the handlebar. Peddle slowly keeping both hands on the

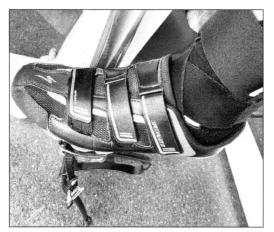

Spin shoe clipped into cleats

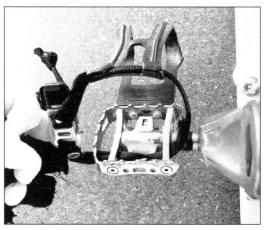

Peddle cleat and basket assembly

handlebar, and adjust the incline/resistance so that you can comfortably reach a cadence rate of 80 RPM (revolutions per minute) or so, as seen at right on the top line of the Keiser display. If 80 RPMs is too fast, try to reach 60 RPM by adjusting the incline/resistance making it lower (easier) if necessary, to comfortably maintain your RPM level. Use this "setting" as your base setting. There you go . . . you're spinning!

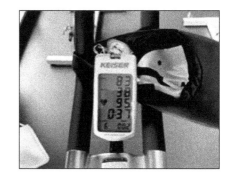

RPM Display (top number)

Final Adjustments

Now, before continuing on to spin session basics, take a minute to make any final adjustments to the seat position, the handlebar, and, if necessary, re-level the bike if you've discovered that it's rocking. Once you've completed any adjustments, remount the bike and again start to slowly turn the peddles using a low incline/resistance setting (e.g., 7 of 30). It's a good idea at this point to familiarize yourself with the incline/resistance control knob/lever while turning the peddles and increasing/decreasing the setting to get a feel for this adjustment, as this can vary quite a bit from one bike to another, even where the spin bike model is the same.

BASIC POSITIONS AND MOVES

Basic spin positions involve the hands and whether you are seated in the saddle or out of the saddle in the standing or extended positions as seen below in this section.

Positions

In your base position, you are seated and relaxed with both hands comfortably on the handlebars as seen below in the "Seated Normal" illustration. You are turning the peddles/flywheel at a cadence rate of 60–80 RPM and the incline/resistance is flat/easy (e.g., 7 of 30). The base position is where you will start and end your sessions and also return to periodically during your spin session—i.e., during the session you will return to the base position during recovery to bring your heart rate down and rehydrate.

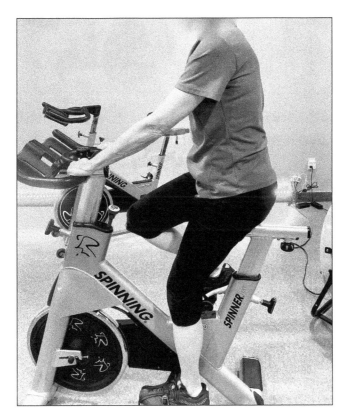

Seated Normal
position

Note the seated hand positions in the two illustrations below, which are out and extended.

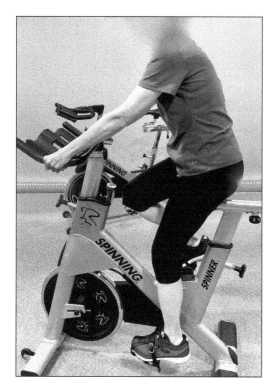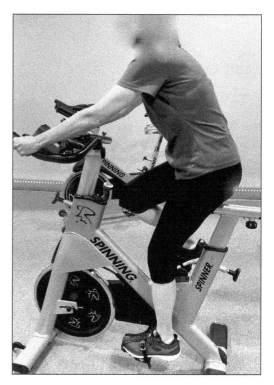

Seated Arms Out and Arms Extended

Finally, see the rider "out of the saddle" in the illustrations on the facing page, again in different hand positions.

Try moving between a few of these positions before returning to the seated base position with the 80 or 60 RPM cadence you established earlier. Keep one hand on the handlebars at all times as you move between positions and change hand positions from normal, out, and extended, as discussed and pictured.

Moves involve moving yourself from one position on the bike to another while either maintaining or intensifying effort by increasing cadence and/or incline/resistance, and also when coming to the rest period, which we refer to as recovery.

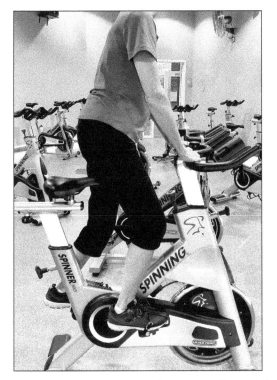 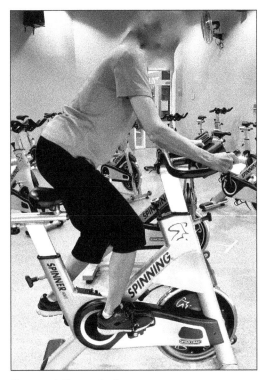

Out of the Saddle Standing and Extended

A sequence of *moves* over a defined period of time makeup a *segment* of the spin session. Taken together, ***positions, moves,*** *and* ***segments*** are the building blocks we'll use to structure YOUR Structured Spinning session in the next chapter.

Moves and Segments

Busting a move isn't just something you do on the dance floor. Moves in spinning are reminiscent of what you see athletes doing during the Tour de France and/ or cyclists challenging themselves in places like the Green Mountains of Vermont. Moves in spinning can be defined as a change in intensity, driven by one or more changes of position, cadence, and/or incline/resistance.

Correspondingly, this change in intensity results in a change in heart rate as you challenge yourself through the session. Just as the cyclist is challenged by a hill in

Vermont, you challenge yourself during a spin session through a series of moves. Furthermore, several moves performed over a prescribed period of time is referred to as a segment. A series of segments over your session time creates the framework for structuring your spin session, which we'll pull together by adding in additional elements in Chapter 4: Structured Spinning. Right now, let's look at the basic moves you'll want to become familiar with.

Starting from *your* base position (e.g., seated, 60–80 RPM, flat/easy incline), here are the basic moves used in spinning.

Jump(s)

This move is performed simply by coming out of the saddle from your base seated position for an 8 count, to either a standing position, or to an out extended position with your butt raised just above the saddle as illustrated in the sequence below. Your hands are either where they were in the base position if standing, or extended. Once out of the saddle, remain out of the saddle while continuing to turn the peddles for an 8-second count before returning to the seated base position for 8 seconds before jumping out of the saddle again for another 8 seconds. The series of jumps in and out of the saddle are repeated for the duration of the segment (e.g., 4 minutes), before recovery (discussed below).

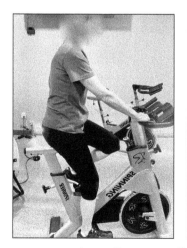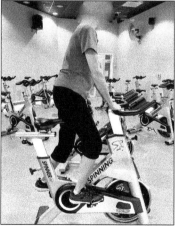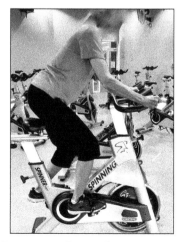

Jump Sequence: Seated to Standing position (and return to Seated)

You can perform this move more aggressively by accelerating your cadence to 90, 100, or higher RPM as you come out of the saddle.

I typically use a segment of standing jumps at the beginning of my spin session as a warm-up, and another segment of jumps at the end to cool down. I'll also use a more intense segment of jumps during the workout portion of my session to elevate my heart rate and challenge myself.

Be careful to monitor the impact of this move on your knees and adjust the number of jumps, segment duration, incline/resistance, etc., if you discover soreness, tightness, or any discomfort, especially later in the day or the following day. Consider using another move in place of jumps if the move bothers your knees. Stretching (discussed in a later chapter) and/or knee supports or ice/cold packs may help.

Standing (and Seated) Incline

This move is performed by adjusting incline/resistance higher while out of the saddle in the standing position as illustrated at right with a normal/flat hand position.

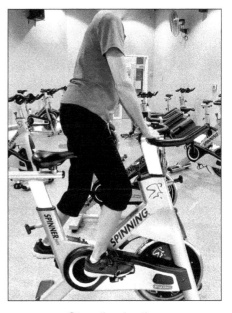

This move is moderately aggressive, as the standing position is maintained for the entire duration of the segment (e.g., 4 minutes) as if jogging uphill on a gentle 5% grade. You raise incline/resistance from the flat base setting to a sustainable moderate setting maintaining a cadence of 50 RPM. During my session, I'll perform a segment of this move to elevate my heart rate to a level approximately 20% higher than that during jumps.

Standing Incline

You can make this move more aggressive by slightly increasing the incline/resistance periodically over the duration of a 4-minute segment—i.e., every 30–60 seconds.

Another way to make this move more aggressive is to perform the segment in the seated position and increase incline/resistance periodically. In either case, you will challenge yourself, and you should see a marked change in heart rate as compared to executing the standing incline move.

Running Up the Hill

Similar but designed to be more aggressive than the previous move, running up the hill requires the rider to increase incline/resistance to an appropriately challenging level while coming out of the saddle to either a standing position or extended position, and accelerating cadence for a defined period of time—e.g., 30 seconds—as if running up a hill with a 10–15% or higher gradient. At the end of the 30 seconds, the rider remains out of the saddle while maintaining the same incline/resistance and decelerates cadence for a defined period before again accelerating cadence for another 30 seconds. Incline/resistance remains the same throughout the segment as the move is repeated for the duration of the segment.

Running up the hill is an aggressive move, especially when performed in the extended position. I often use this move to "max out" my heart rate, by reaching my maximum *targeted* heart rate for the session—i.e., 85% of my age-adjusted maximum heart rate. You can make this move even more aggressive by flattening your back and projecting your chest and upper body forward over the handlebars.

While this move should not be taken lightly, even the newest of spinning disciples can work in the move by adjusting incline/resistance, cadence, and durations while monitoring heart rate through the segment.

Sprints

As the name implies, a sprint in spinning is to peddle very fast for a defined period—e.g., execute a high cadence level of 110 RPM (or higher) for a period of 40 seconds. Sprints are usually performed in the saddle and are often accompanied by an increased level of incline/resistance. The sprint is held for a defined period before returning to your base RPM for a period of 30–60 seconds, and then the sprint is repeated for another 40 seconds. The move is done repeatedly for the duration of the segment.

A more aggressive sprint is started by coming out of the saddle for a 5 count to reach the targeted (110) RPM after increasing incline/resistance, and then returning to the saddle and maintaining the 110 RPM for the remainder of the move. In this case, the rider is challenged to perform the move with higher incline/resistance by coming out of the saddle for the initial 5 count, and then maintaining the 110 RPM at the higher incline/resistance for the duration.

Sprints are a good move to work into different parts of a session to quickly change/ regulate heart rate to a desired level. I use sprints in both early and late parts of my workout to "regulate" my heart rate on the upside of the session as I work toward maximum heart rate, and on the cooldown side of my session to make sure I don't cool down too fast. They are an important move in supporting Structured Spinning.

Recovery

A recovery period follows each segment of each of the above moves, whereby you return to your base seated position and RPM. For example, after a 4-minute segment of "running up the hill," you should allow your heart and muscles to recover at a comfortable BPM by returning to the base position and rehydrating. Over the course of your spin session, this form of *active* recovery prevents a post-exercise drop in blood pressure to the brain by enhancing the flow of blood back to the heart, increasing cardiac stroke volume and output.

A 60-second recovery between segments allows your heart to return to a resting rate of 80–90 BPM and enables you to continue your workout safely while continuing to challenge yourself and reach your goals for the session. Recovery times should be adjusted based on your level of fitness and be thought of as an enabling feature of the session. Also, near the end of each session, you will use a recovery segment to "cool down" and lower your heart rate before getting off the bike to stretch. I'll discuss recovery-cooldown-stretch as part of Structured Spinning in the next chapter.

CHAPTER 3 SUMMARY

This chapter discusses the basics of spinning by first introducing two additional elements—incline/resistance and cadence—before proceeding with setting up the bike prior to the rider mounting it and beginning to spin. The setup discussion includes leveling the bike, handlebar and seat adjustments, peddles, shoes, and mounting the bike. The chapter then discusses and illustrates positions and basic moves/segments, including recovery.

CHAPTER 4

Structured Spinning

So, what is Structured Spinning? It's my own personal spinning methodology that measures and controls each of the components of spinning discussed in the prior chapter—i.e., time and duration, incline/resistance, cadence, and most importantly, heart rate. Each of these is monitored during your spin session as you execute moves and segments. By monitoring and measuring each component throughout the ride, we provide ourselves with a repeatable, self-motivating method for attaining and maintaining physical conditioning and goals. Unlike attending spin classes that vary greatly without purpose or direction from one day to the next, Structured Spinning sessions ultimately are designed by you to reflect both your condition from day to day, as well as supporting your long-term conditioning goals related to weight, muscle tone, and strength. Each day you spin, every session is truly *YOUR RIDE*!

Keeping the personalized design of Structured Spinning in mind, I'm going to discuss the basic structure of a Structured Spinning session, review the basic elements we use to measure and achieve degrees of intensity and difficulty, and then demonstrate this in a 30-minute Structured Spinning workout. All the Structured Spinning session workouts in this guide are yours to use; however, it's important to keep in mind that it's my intention that you will eventually construct Structured Spinning sessions tailored to your own condition, goals, and liking.

BASICS OF STRUCTURED SPINNING

So let's get to it! The basic structure of *every* Structured Spinning session includes:

1. Pre-ride stretch

2. Warmup

3. The challenge

4. Cooldown

5. Post-ride stretch

You'll find some semblance of this structure in the fitness club spin classes; however, there typically is no consistency or sense of repeatability between sessions, and some instructors skim through or bypass sections entirely. In any case, the important stuff is in the detailed structure of each part—i.e., the moves/segments, time/duration, heart rate (as beats per minute; BPM), cadence (RPM), and incline/resistance, throughout every spin session. Let's take a closer look and examine a simple 30-minute session, timed from when you sit on the bike and begin to turn the pedals till you dismount the bike. But first, let's get ready to ride with a quick stretch.

Pre-ride Stretch

Before starting any ride, you should perform a short stretch once the bike has been setup (see "Before Getting on the Bike" in Chapter 3 if you have not yet set up your bike). My pre-ride stretch is quick and easy, executed in under 5 minutes, and includes the following in this order:

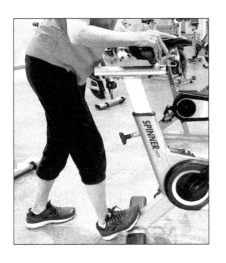

Calf Stretch

Stand behind the bike and place one foot a time against the back frame of the bike (as shown at left). Using the seat, pull yourself slowly and gently in toward the seat as illustrated. Feel the calf muscles and Achilles tendon stretch, and hold the stretch for 10–15 seconds. Do the same with the opposite foot before continuing to the next stretch: back rotations.

Back Rotation

Standing to either side of the bike and anchoring the edge of one or both feet slightly under the bike frame for support, bring your fists into your chest with your elbows pointed outward, and gently rotate your upper body to the right, and then back to center. Then rotate your upper body to the left and back to center. Repeat this rotating motion for 8–10 seconds, feeling the lower back loosen. See the sequence of images below.

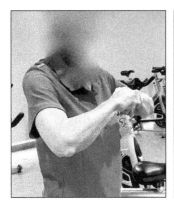 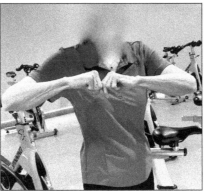 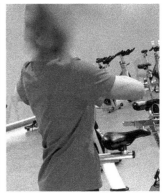

Back Rotation

Side Stretch

Standing at arm's length to either side of the bike, place your left hand out to grasp the seat while moving your left foot out in front of your right foot. Now move your right arm up, reaching high above your head and toward the seat while bending your upper body toward the bike seat. Feel the stretch in your right-side muscles; now, try moving your arm and head further in the direction of the seat, slowly increasing the stretch. You're doing this correctly when the stretch is felt into the right hip and leg. Execute the stretch for 10–15 seconds; when done, execute another 8–10-second series of back rotations before performing the side stretch on the other side. Repeat another 8–10-second series of back rotations before continuing to the next stretch.

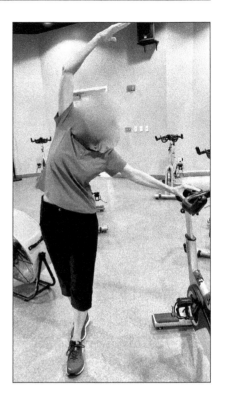

Quad Stretch

Standing on the right side of the bike facing forward, place your left hand on the seat to steady yourself while reaching behind you with the other hand to gently pull your right foot and leg up behind your butt, as illustrated in the left-hand image on the facing page. Hold the position for 5–8 seconds and try to pull your leg further upward toward the sky. Use your leg muscles to push the leg up and back while your hand pulls in the same direction. Bend forward lowering your head while stretching the leg upward and to the side (facing page, right). Hold this position for another 5 seconds while feeling your quadricep and inner thigh stretch. Slowly return to the standing position while releasing the leg from your hand.

When done, execute another 8–10-second series of back rotations before performing the quad stretch on the other side, positioning yourself on either side of the bike to stretch your other quadricep. When done, repeat another 8–10-second series of back rotations before continuing to the next stretch.

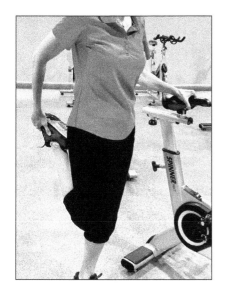 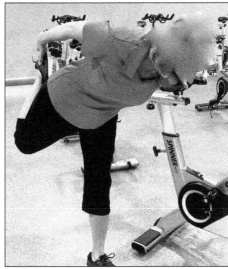

Quad
Stretch

Hamstring Stretch

Facing to the rear of the bike from the right side, hold the handlebar with your right hand and raise your left foot up to rest the back of the heel on the seat of the bike as seen below. Use your left hand to help raise your leg if necessary. Alternatively, if you find it difficult to raise your foot to rest on the seat, bring it to the bike's crossbar of the frame as shown in the center picture below. Now with the leg elevated, gently flatten the extended leg and move both hands to the shin below the knee and reach toward the foot and toes while lowering and moving your head forward toward your knee. Feel the upper posterior hamstring muscle stretch. Hold the stretch for a count of 8 and then slowly turn your upper body toward the leg anchored on the floor while reaching toward the foot and bend your knee to touch your foot. Feel the stretch deep in the groin to a count of 5 before returning your upper body to the extended leg and foot resting on the seat.

Hold the stretch as pictured for a 5 count before relaxing it and returning your right hand to the handlebar before moving your leg from the seat, using your left hand to assist if necessary. Come to a standing position. Execute another series of back rotations before positioning yourself to stretch the left leg. When done, repeat another series of back rotations.

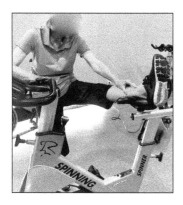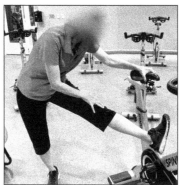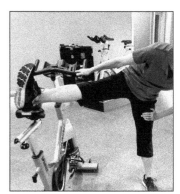

Hamstring Stretch

Note: While your foot is elevated on the seat and hands are forward, ensure that your spin shoe straps are comfortably tight.

Warmup Segment (5 minutes)

Now that the Pre-ride stretches are done, let's move on to the warmup segment. The purpose of the warmup segment is to increase blood flow primarily to the leg muscles. To accomplish this, you'll need to elevate your heart rate from its resting rate, which is typically 45–49% of your maximum heart rate, to your base rate of approximately 60% of maximum heart rate.

Each person's base will be different, but a reasonable target to begin with is a heart rate of 60–65% of your maximum heart rate. To determine your maximum heart rate, the Mayo Clinic says to subtract your age from 220—e.g., if you're 50 years old, your maximum heart rate is calculated as 220 - 50 = 170. Therefore, your base rate, 60–65% of maximum, is between 102–110 BPM (between 170 x 60% and 170 x 65%).

So, in the warmup segment, you will elevate your heart rate from its resting rate (70+/-) to your base heart rate. To do this, start by raising the rate you are peddling to 80 revolutions per minute (RPM), and apply a light incline/resistance setting to the flywheel. On the Keiser bike shown in Chapter 2, this would be an incline/

resistance level setting of around 6 or 7 (out of 30) . . . pretty light. It may take a few minutes the first time you try it, but if you play around with the incline/resistance and RPM, you will find a comfortable level of effort that you feel you can maintain indefinitely at a heart rate equal to 60–65% of your maximum.

So let's try it and start spinning! Mount the bike and clip in your shoes or position them into the pedal baskets. Begin turning the pedals, adding a small amount of incline/resistance and start timing this 5-minute warmup segment. For the next 5 minutes, you'll elevate your heart rate to its base level and warm up the muscles of your body to get ready to challenge yourself from your base level.

The base level of your workout structure is what you'll warm up to in this initial segment, and, later in the session, the base level is where you'll return to after each segment of the challenge portion of your workout to allow your body to recover before starting another challenge segment. Your base level is defined by the incline/resistance level, and cadence/RPM level that support a comfortable target heart rate (e.g., 60% of maximum heart rate) for a desired period of time/duration, which in this case is for the 5-minute warmup segment. At the end of the warmup segment, you'll move on to the first segment of the 20-minute challenge portion of this 30-minute ride.

The Challenge (20 minutes)

The challenge portion of the session is where you execute the most rigorous and strenuous segments of the session. It should be focused toward achieving your goal for the day's session. Your goal for the day may be to burn a target number of calories or maybe to reach and hold a target heart rate for an extended period, or a combination of both. Or perhaps you will want to strengthen a muscle group like the quads for a certain period and thereby design the segments of the challenge portion of your workout to include moves that focus on the quad muscles. Over time, as you become more acquainted with the methodology, the goals and objectives you set for yourself will become self-evident and fulfilling.

For example, in this basic 30-minute session, I will achieve a 350-calorie burn; increase and hold my heart rate at a mid-70% of maximum BPM range for a period, before topping out at 83% of maximum BPM. I will achieve my heart rate objectives over the next four segments of the challenge, executed over a 20-minute period starting immediately after the warmup.

First Segment: 8-Second Jumps (4 minutes)

As you finish the warmup segment, increase incline/resistance sightly—e.g., on the Keiser bike, raise the incline/resistance from the warmup level of 6, to 8 or 9 and execute an 8-second jump (see "Moves and Segments" in Chapter 3) by coming out of the saddle and maintaining a comfortable RPM. After an 8 count, lower yourself back to the saddle and increase cadence to your Base RPM of 80 for an 8 count. Then repeat the jump again and continue the 8-second jump sequence for the 4-minute duration. Your heart rate will fluctuate between 67–73% of maximum as you jump out and return to the saddle throughout the duration of the segment. At the end of the 4 minutes, return to the saddle and execute a 1-minute recovery.

*Recovery–*1 minute in the saddle at your base level to recover from the 4-minute jump segment. It's important to *hydrate* during every recovery period and observe your heart rate as it returns toward your base heart rate BPM. The quickness in which it takes your heart rate to return to your base BPM is a good indication of your cardio condition. Over time, as you improve your conditioning, you'll notice that your heart rate returns more quickly to the base BPM rate during recovery.

Second Segment: Standing Incline (4 minutes)

As your 1-minute recovery nears an end, increase the incline/resistance slightly (e.g., on the Keiser bike, increase the incline/resistance from your base of 6, to 8 or 9) and come out of the saddle to a standing position while lowering your cadence to 50–60 RPMs (see "Moves and Segments" in Chapter 3). This segment is intended to resemble having an easy jog. Maintain this jog for the 4-minute segment and observe your heart rate as it increases by 20% from the recovery to 72–74% of your maximum BPM. Adjust incline/resistance and cadence to achieve and maintain this heart rate level. At the end of this 4-minute segment, return to the saddle and execute a 1-minute recovery.

Recovery–1 minute in the saddle at your base level to recover. It's important to *hydrate* during every recovery period and observe your heart rate as it returns toward your base BPM. The quickness in which it takes your heart rate to return to your base BPM is a good indication of your cardio condition.

Third Segment–Running Up the Hill (4 minutes)

This segment is designed to elevate your heart rate to 80–83% of your maximum BPM. Throughout the 4-minute segment, you will maintain a rate above 69% of your maximum heart rate.

As your 1-minute recovery from the second segment nears an end, increase the incline/resistance moderately (e.g., on the Keiser bike increase the incline/resistance from your base of 6, to 9 or 10) and come out of the saddle to a standing position, simultaneously increasing your cadence to 90–100 RPMs, as if you were running up a hill (see "Moves and Segments" in Chapter 3). Maintain this cadence for 30 seconds, and observe your heart rate as it jumps to 73–75% of your maximum BPM. Adjust incline/resistance and cadence to achieve and maintain this heart rate level.

At the end of the 30-second run, remain in the standing position and reduce your cadence to a comfortable 50–60 RPM jog for 40 seconds as you observe your heart rate as it falls; then, accelerate your cadence again to run up the hill for the second 30-second burst. Observe your heart rate jump to 76–79% of your maximum BPM. Adjust incline/resistance and cadence to achieve and maintain this heart rate level while in the second run. At the end of the second run, remain in the standing position and reduce your cadence to a comfortable 50–60 RPM jog for 40 seconds. Repeat the 30-second run up the hill two more times, returning to the saddle after the fourth and final burst. Observe your heart rate as it jumps to 77–83% of your maximum BPM during these last two runs. Adjust incline/resistance and cadence to achieve and maintain this heart rate level. At the end of the last run up the hill, return to the saddle for a 1-minute recovery.

Recovery–1 minute in the saddle at your base level. It's important to *hydrate* during every recovery period and observe your heart rate as it returns toward your Base BPM. The quickness in which it takes your heart rate to return to your base BPM is a good indication of your cardio condition.

Fourth Segment–Running Jumps (4 minutes)

This segment is designed to be a working cooldown from the previous segment, as you continue this fourth segment at a more moderate level for the next 4 minutes, during which you will elevate and maintain your heart rate from your base level in recovery to 74–77% of your maximum BPM.

As your 1-minute recovery nears an end, increase the incline/resistance sightly—e.g., on the Keiser bike, raise the incline/resistance from your base level of 6, increasing it to 8 or 9 and execute an 8-count jump (see "Moves and Segments" in Chapter 3), coming out of the saddle *and* simultaneously increasing your cadence from base to 95–105 RPM. After being out of the saddle at the higher RPM for an 8-count, lower yourself back to the saddle and return to an RPM of 80 for an 8-count. Repeat the running jump again and continue the 8-count running jumps followed by an 8-count return to the saddle for the duration of the 4-minute segment. Observe your heart rate fluctuating between 74–77% of maximum for the duration. Adjust incline/resistance and cadence to achieve and maintain this heart rate level. At the end of this 4-minute segment, return to the saddle and execute a 1-minute recovery.

Recovery–1 minute in the saddle at your Base level to recover. It's important to *hydrate* during every recovery period and observe your heart rate as it returns toward your base BPM. The quickness in which it takes your heart rate to return to your base BPM is a good indication of your cardio condition.

Cooldown (5 minutes)

The cooldown portion of Structured Spinning is executed in the saddle as you continue to turn the peddles at your base spin level. During the cooldown, we will begin stretching, continue hydrating, and observe our heart rate as it returns toward our resting heart rate and that level observed at the beginning of the warmup—e.g., approximately 60% of maximum BPM. By the end of the 5-minute cooldown, you will have completed the stretches below in under 5 minutes before dismounting the bike and moving on to the post-ride stretch portion of the session. Allow the 5-minute cooldown segment to expire and continue at your base rate once you've completed the stretches, before dismounting.

As your final challenge recovery minute ends, execute the easy stretches below while in the saddle, using an 8-second count as a guide while continuing to move the peddles. Check that you maintain cadence and heart rate at your base level and adjust incline/resistance to support your upper body movements while stretching. If you feel unbalanced or insecure during any of these stretches, try slowing your cadence and/or adjusting incline/resistance. If you're still uncomfortable, keep one hand on the handlebar and try the stretch singlehandedly, alternating hands. Finally, if you are still uncomfortable stretching while on the bike, after a minute or two of letting your heart rate come down to 60%, dismount the bike and perform the stretches while standing on the floor. Hopefully over time you will feel more secure and be able to perform these stretches while continuing to turn the peddles.

That being said, begin each of the following stretches by sitting up straight in the saddle with both hands at your side while maintaining your base spinning level. Remember to hydrate between each stretch.

Shoulder Shrug Rotations—With your arms at your side, raise your shoulders as if trying to touch your ears and rotate your shoulders forward and then down; repeat the shoulder raise and forward rotation several times. Feel the stretch in your shoulders as you continue to rotate them for an 8 count. Then execute this same stretch by moving your raised shoulders backward and down several times. Finally, alternate between forward and backward rotations for another 8 count.

Arms Up–Raise both arms up straight above your head (as seen at right), and gently move side to side, stretching your upper body.

Arms Left, Right, and Behind–From the previous stretch position, hold one hand with the other and lower your arms so that they are extended out forward in front of you (see left image below).

Now rotate your upper body slightly to the right, as seen in the center image below, and feel the stretch in your left shoulder and arm for an 8 count. Rotate back to center and continue to rotate slightly left of center, feeling the stretch in your right shoulder and arm for an 8 count before returning to center and releasing your hands to your side.

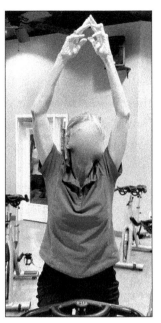

Arms Up

Finally, clasp your hands behind your back and raise them slightly skyward (below, far right). Tilt your upper body slightly forward and continue to raise your arms a little more, feeling the stretch in your shoulder for an 8 count. Slowly lower your arms and release your hands, returning them to your side as you continue to turn the peddles at your base spin rate and hydrate while moving on to the next stretch.

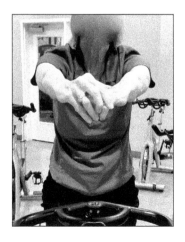
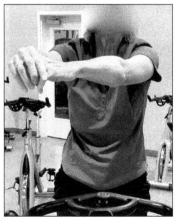
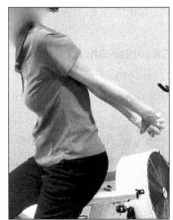

Lateral Shoulder Rotations–
Raise your arms from your side to point them outward horizontally with your thumbs pointing up, as pictured at right. With both arms, make small 12-inch circles while your arms are extended outward and thumbs up. After an 8 count, reverse the direction

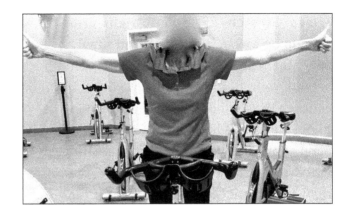

of your hands to circle to the back with the thumbs still pointing up. After an 8 count, turn your hand so your thumbs are pointing down, and reverse the direction of your circling hands two more times, circling each for 8 counts. Remember to continue to turn the peddles at your base spin rate as you perform the lateral shoulder rotations and hydrate before moving on to the next stretch.

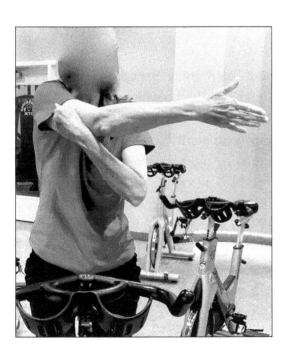

Shoulder Stretch–Move your right arm across your chest and support it with your left wrist and forearm as illustrated at left. *Gently* straighten the extended right arm to the left while turning your head to look over your right shoulder. Hold this position for an 8 count before slowly releasing it to return your arm to your right side, and bring your head forward. Switching sides, perform this shoulder stretch with the left arm stretched across your chest to the right, supporting it with the right forearm for an 8 count, with your eyes looking left.

Tricep Stretch–Raise your right arm straight up toward the ceiling and slowly bend the arm at your elbow to reach behind your head, touching your back between the shoulder blades as shown in the picture at right. With your opposite hand, hold the bent elbow and gently move the right arm lower, feeling the right tricep stretch. Hold the stretch for an 8 count before releasing your elbow and moving your right arm to your side. Remember to continue to turn the peddles at your base spin rate as you perform the stretches and hydrate while moving on to the next stretch.

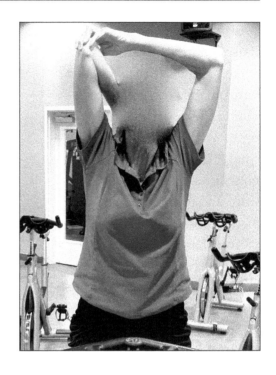

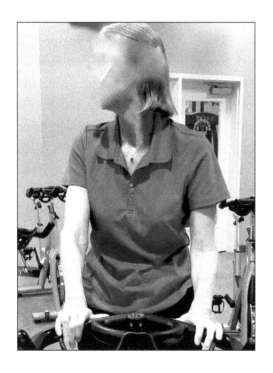

Head Turn Neck Stretch–Perform this stretch while holding the handlebars. Start by simply looking forward and turn your head gently to the right looking out over your right shoulder; then, turn your head back to center before turning to the left and looking out over your left shoulder, before returning your gaze forward. Slowly repeat the right-center-left-center head turn several times, feeling the side neck muscles stretching. Continue for an 8 count.

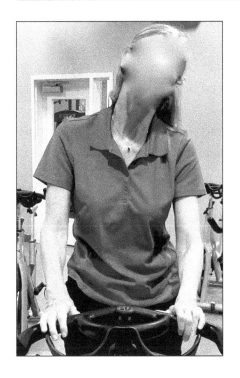

Neck Bend Stretch–Perform this stretch while holding the handlebars. Start by simply looking forward and slowly lower your head, dropping it downward toward and touching your chin to your chest. Ease into the stretch and feel the back of your neck loosen and stretch. Hold this position for an 8 count. Now with your head still lowered, roll it toward your right as if trying to touch your right ear to your right shoulder, and then slowly move your head up and down as if signaling "yes" to the person on your right. Perform this up-and-down head movement while turned to the right for an 8 count before slowly raising your head to return your gaze back to center, looking straight out. Repeat the stretch on the left side.

Neck Roll Rotation Stretch–Perform this stretch while holding the handlebars. Start by simply looking forward and slowly lower your head and touch your chin to your chest. With your chin touching your chest, slowly begin to roll your head toward your right shoulder before looking right out over your shoulder, and continue to roll your head right and toward the ceiling, eventually looking upward. Continue now rolling your head toward the left shoulder before returning your chin to center on your chest. Perform two of these rotations to the right before coming to center and starting the same neck rotations to the left. Repeat alternating rotations slowly, each for at least an 8 count before performing another set of the "Neck Bend Stretches" above. Remember to continue to turn the peddles at your base spin rate as you perform the stretches and hydrate while moving on to the next stretch.

Dismounting and Post-ride Stretch

During the preceding cooldown segment of the session, we stretched the upper portion of the body, continued to hydrate, and observed our heart rate return toward a resting heart rate level—i.e., approximately 58–61% of maximum. Now before dismounting the bike, reduce your peddle speed and slowly come to a stop (apply incline/resistance if necessary), with both feet parallel and equally distanced to the floor with one foot forward and one foot back. Keep your feet in this position and raise yourself out of the saddle to stand on the peddles, as illustrated below. Remain in this standing position on the peddles and slowly let your heels drop lower than the toes to stretch the Achilles tendon and calf. Hold this stretch for an 8 count. If you are more comfortable doing this one foot at a time, then lower one heel at a time while the opposite foot stays flat on the peddle. Then stretch the opposite side.

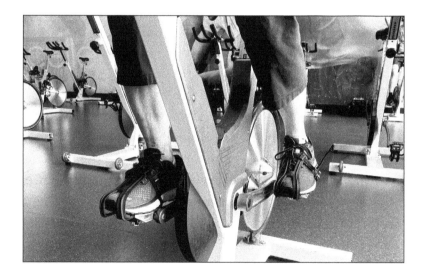

Continue to observe your heart rate while executing this stretch and remain in the standing position on the bike until your heart rate is below 62% of maximum. Then release one foot at a time from the peddle clip or remove one foot at a time from its basket to the floor, and come to a standing position next to the bike. Continue to hydrate before and during the following floor stretches.

The post-ride floor stretches include all five of the pre-ride stretches described earlier, plus additional calf, hip, and side stretches. The pre-ride stretches to be done as part of the post-ride stretch are calf stretch, back rotation, side stretch, quad stretch, and hamstring. Execute each of the five pre-ride stretches, augmenting each calf stretch with calf raises as described below. Once you've completed the pre-ride stretches, continue with the hip, back, and side stretches described below. Remember to continue to hydrate and perform back rotations in between each stretch.

Calf Raises–Each calf stretch should be followed by 20 calf raises, as illustrated below. Start by moving to either the side or to the rear of the bike and placing the front of the sole of one foot onto the flat portion of the bike frame. The heel of the foot remains on the floor, as shown below.

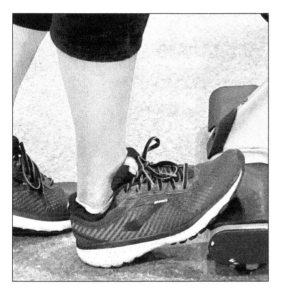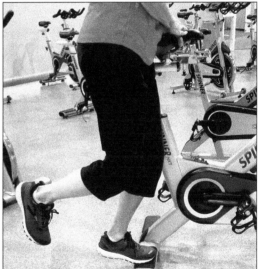

Now bring your hands to the bike seat for balance (shown above, at right) and raise your body up as much as possible using only the calf muscle of the foot whose sole is on the bike frame. Use your hands to maintain balance and resist the urge to use them to assist the calf in raising your body.

After a second, lower yourself to the starting position, and then elevate yourself again repeating the calf raise. Perform 20 calf raises before switching to the other foot and performing 20 calf raises on the second foot. If you find it difficult to perform 20 calf raises as described above, push up from the seat with your hands to assist the calf muscles.

Now complete the remaining four pre-ride stretches before continuing on to the post-ride stretches below. Remember to hydrate and perform back rotations between each stretch.

Hip Stretches–I use two positions to stretch the hips after *every* ride. They are performed in sequence; the first being in a single leg sit-like position, and the second, a bent knee hip stretch.

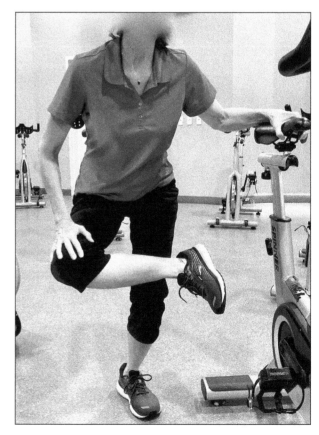

To reach the single leg sit-like position, you will use the bike for support by holding the seat as shown at right. Be careful not to place too much weight on the seat or the bike will tip and/or slide toward you.

Begin by standing on the right side of the bike facing forward or toward the seat, and grasp either the handlebar or seat with your left hand for support. Very slowly bend your knees and lower your body as if you were going to sit on a chair. As you lower your torso use your right hand to assist in raising your right ankle, resting it on your left knee and coming to a seat-like position as illustrated. *Be careful* not to place too much weight on the seat or handlebars or the bike will tip and/or slide toward you.

Once you've reached the seated position, rest your free right hand on the elevated right knee and gently push it downward, feeling the stretch in your right hip. Hold the stretch for an 8 count before releasing it; and then, using your right hand, support your right ankle as it slides away from your knee, returning your right foot to the floor while coming to a standing position to perform a bent-knee hip stretch.

Begin the bent-knee hip stretch by facing to the front from the right side of the bike and placing your left hand on the seat for support. Move your left foot a step forward and the right foot toward the rear while slowly lowering yourself and further extending the right leg as far to the rear as is comfortable, coming to rest on your right toe. Continue to lower your torso while bending the left knee and extending the right leg so the right knee is near to or briefly touches the floor. Feel the right hip stretch and hold this position for an 8 count before raising yourself up to a standing position.

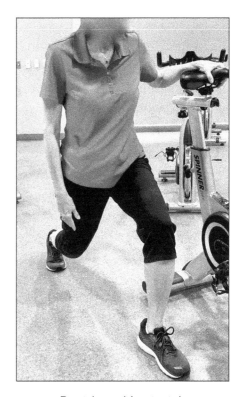

Also, you may find it more comfortable extending the left leg back instead of the right leg. Either way works just as well so use whichever way feels most comfortable.

Bent-knee hip stretch

Now perform both hip stretches on the opposite side. Perform back rotations and hydrate before moving on to the final set of back stretches.

Back Stretches–I use three positions with back stretches. Once you've completed them, you've completed the spin session. While these back stretches are relatively benign, it is important to consider the condition of your back before executing them. The back stretches are performed in series: backward lean, upward reaches, and side reaches.

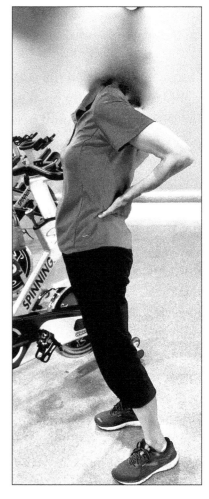

As with back rotations, the backward lean is best performed by finding a place on the bottom of the bike frame where it meets the floor, where you are able to slightly insert the side of your foot or toe in between the floor and frame. By doing so, it will support your body weight and allow you to maximize the backward lean stretch and help you from falling backward and having to step back to catch yourself.

Once you've found a point between the floor and the bike to place your foot, take a comfortable stance with your feet spread at shoulder width, and support your back by placing your hands on the lower portion of your back as shown below, and look up to the ceiling, slowly letting your shoulders drift to the rear. Be sure to have your hands on your lower back for support as your upper torso drifts back as far as is comfortable without coming out of the stance.

Hold the position for an 8 count, feeling the stretch in the lower and middle back muscles. Return to the starting position, and while your foot is still between the floor and bike frame, execute a series of back rotations. Once done, hydrate before moving on to perform upward reaches.

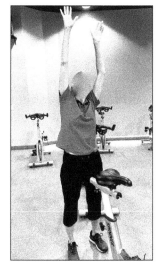

Upward reaches

Upward reaches are very simple moves to provide additional stretches of your side and back muscles. From the standing position with legs separated at shoulder width, look to the ceiling and extend your arms up extending one arm at a time to reach upward as much as is comfortable. Perform these reaches alternating arms for an 8 count and move directly to side stretches.

Side Stretches are done with your arms still reaching skyward and maintaining the same foot stance. Hold the fingers of one hand with the other and rotate your torso to the right, feeling the stretch in the left arm, shoulder, and side into the trap (trapezius) and lat (latissimus) muscles. Hold the position for an 8 count before returning to center, and then rotate your torso to extend to the left, repeating the stretch on the opposite side for another 8 count. It's important in this stretch to maintain your foot stance, but don't overdo the rotation; rotate only as much as is comfortable.

Come back to center with the arms still reaching to the sky. Then release your hands and again perform upward reaches. Hydrate, and *you're done!*

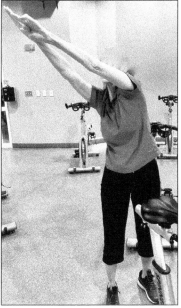

Side stretches

CHAPTER 4 SUMMARY

In this chapter the primary structural components that make up every Structured Spinning session are covered, and the Structured Spinning methodology is illustrated using a simple 30-minute spin session. The components of a Structured Spinning session include pre-ride stretch, warm-up, the challenge, cooldown, and post-ride stretch. The 30-minute ride includes segments/moves such as jumps, running up the hill, sprints, and running jumps, illustrating targeted heart rates (BPM), cadence, and incline/resistance for defined durations. A variety of stretches, both on the bike and from the floor, are discussed and photo illustrated.

CHAPTER 5

More Structured Spinning Workouts

The 30-minute Structured Spinning session illustrated in Chapter 4 is a handy workout for many adopters of Structured Spinning. New riders will find it to be a comfortable ride that they can adjust and adapt to by making it more or less challenging as desired based on current conditioning. Also, if your workouts include weightlifting, yoga, or other classes, a 30-minute cardio workout that also includes stretching is not too time consuming to include in your regular workout. After all, most of us don't find the time to allocate much more than 90 minutes in the gym on any given day, so this 30-minute spin may be just what the doctor ordered.

So, while 30-minute spins allow time for other strength-building exercises, for many years my Structured Spinning sessions were 60 minutes, or sometimes 45 minutes if my gym time was limited. Again, you'll want to make it your ride; so, in this chapter I'll illustrate a 60-minute ride and show you a table graphic you can use to design your own Structured Spinning session.

60-MINUTE STRUCTURED SPINNING SESSION

The basic structure of *every* Structured Spinning session includes 1) pre-ride Stretch, 2) warm-up, 3) the challenge, 4) cooldown, and 5) post-ride stretch. The same structure applies regardless of whether it's a 30-, 45-, 60-, or 90-minute spin, or whatever time you are allocating to your spin session. What changes is the challenge portion of the session, which is longer and includes more segments and moves designed to support the day's workout target(s) and your longer-term health/fitness needs and goals.

In my 60-minute session, the challenge portion includes all the segments/moves illustrated in Chapter 4, and brings in both seated and standing climbs, sprints, and running jumps. The challenge portion of the 60-minute session is performed after the same pre-ride stretch and warm-up and is followed by the cooldown and post-ride stretch (again, see Chapter 4).

The following chart illustrates the 60-minute session. Also, a blank chart is included in the appendix, which can be used to design your own sessions. Request a PDF of this chart by emailing me at Structured_Spinning@Yahoo.com.

Several of the moves below were not in the preceding chapter's 30-minute spin session. These additional moves are described below the chart and include standing incline, seated incline, sprints, and running jumps.

Segment	Move	Hands/ Position	Duration	Incline/ Resistance	Cadence/ RPM	Heart Rate/BPM
1. Warm-up	Base level	Flat/Seated	5 minutes	Flat / 7 of 30 (Base)	80 RPMs (Base)	60% of max (Base)
2. Challenge	8 Second Jumps	Choice/Up-Seated	4 minutes	Gentle / 9 of 30	80 RPMs seated, 60 RPMs up	67%–73%
3. Challenge	Recovery	Flat/Seated	1 minute	Flat / 7 of 30	Base	Base
4. Challenge	Standing Jog	Choice/Up	4 minutes	Gentle / 9 of 30	50–60 RPMs	72%–74%
5. Challenge	Recovery	Flat/Seated	1 minute	Flat / 7 of 30	Base	Base
6. Challenge	30 Second Runs Up the Hill	Choice/Up	4 minutes	Uphill / 11 of 30	90–100 RPMs	73%–83%

Segment	Move	Hands/Position	Duration	Incline/Resistance	Cadence/RPM	Heart Rate/BPM
7. Challenge	Recovery	Flat/Seated	1 minute	Flat / 7 of 30	Base	Base
8. Challenge	8 Second Jumps	Choice/Up-Seated	4 minutes	Gentle / 9 of 30	80 RPMs seated, 60 RPMs up	67%–73%
9. Challenge	Recovery	Flat/Seated	1 minute	Flat / 7 of 30	Base	Base
10. Challenge	Standing Incline	Choice/Up	4 minutes	Uphill / 11–14 of 30	50–60 RPMs	74%–83%
11. Challenge	Recovery	Flat/Seated	1 minute	Flat / 7 of 30	Base	Base
12. Challenge	8 Second Jumps	Choice/Up-Seated	4 minutes	Uphill / 11 of 30	80 RPMs seated, 60 RPMs up	67%–73%
13. Challenge	Recovery	Flat/Seated	1 minute	Flat / 7 of 30	Base	Base
14. Challenge	Seated Incline	Flat	4 minutes	Steep / 13–15 of 30	40–60 RPMs	73%–83%
15. Challenge	Recovery	Flat/Seated	1 minute	Flat / 7 of 30	Base	Base
16. Challenge	Sprints	Flat/Seated	4 minutes	Elevating 9 to 12	110–120 RPMs	73%–83%
17. Challenge	Recovery	Flat/Seated	1 minute	Flat / 7 of 30	Base	Base
18. Challenge	Running Jumps	Choice/Up	4 minutes	Gentle / 9 of 30	80 RPMs seated, 100 RPMs up	72%–79%
19. Challenge	Recovery	Flat/Seated	1 minute	Flat / 7 of 30	Base	Base
20. Challenge	Standing Jog	Choice/Up	4 minutes	Gentle / 9 of 30	50–60 RPMs	72%–74%
21. Challenge	Recovery	Flat/Seated	1 minute	Flat / 7 of 30	Base	Base
22. Cool-down	Base level - Stretches	Flat/Seated	5 minutes	Flat / 7 of 30 (Base)	80 RPMs (Base)	60% of max (Base)

60-Minute Session Challenge (50 minutes)

The challenge portion of the 60-minute session is 50 minutes where your heart rate and respiratory system are elevated above 65% and will achieve a maximum rate above 80% several times. It is during this part of your session where you can focus on achieving your goals for the day—i.e., calorie burn, muscle strengthening, heart rate endurance, etc.

During this 60-minute session, I typically burn more than 750 calories and increase my cardiorespiratory endurance by reaching 83% of maximum heart rate during several segments of the challenge portion of the ride. A good deal of this is due to the following additional segments to the 30-minute ride: standing incline, seated incline, sprints, and running jumps.

Standing Incline (4 minutes)

The standing incline is designed to raise your heart rate toward the 80% of max level over the 4 minutes that you are out of the saddle with your hands either flat on the handlebar or extended out if you choose to elevate your butt just slightly off the saddle. The latter form will dramatically increase the workload of your quadriceps; or, if it's your first time, keep your hands flat on the handlebars and come to an upright standing position as if performing the standing jog.

In either case, begin the segment with the incline/resistance set to 11 of 30 and increase incline/resistance one step every minute so that it is 14 during the final minute. Maintain your peddle speed at 50–60 RPMs and at the end of the 4-minute standing incline move, return to the saddle and execute a 1-minute recovery.

Seated Incline (4 minutes)

The seated incline is surprisingly one of the most aggressive moves simply due to its seated position, requiring the legs to do all the work as opposed to the standing incline where your body weight contributes much toward turning the flywheel. The seated incline move requires the legs to do most of the work.

A nice variation of this move is done by periodically elevating your butt slightly from the saddle with hands extended, as if performing a jump, holding this raised position for a period (20 seconds) before returning to the saddle for a period (20 seconds) and then repeating the raised position. Repeating this in-and-out of the saddle move for the 4-minute segment makes the move much more aggressive and is a good way to elevate your spin workout.

To start off with this move, begin the segment with incline/resistance set to 11 of 30 and increase incline/resistance one step every minute so that it is 14 during the final minute. Maintain your peddle speed at 50–60 RPMs during the segment, and at the end of the segment. execute a 1-minute recovery.

Sprints (4 minutes)

Sprints are performed by accelerating from your base cadence of 60–80 RPM to a high-intensity burst reaching and maintaining cadence of 110+ RPM for a duration of 40 seconds.

There are two forms of sprints: in the saddle and starting out of the saddle. There are three moves to the 4-minute segment, where you will accelerate cadence each time to the 110 RPM level.

In the Saddle–To start the first move of an in the saddle segment, increase incline/ resistance from your base of 6 or 7 to 10, and increase your cadence from your base rate of 60–80 RPM quickly to 110 RPM. Maintain this elevated RPM for 40 seconds. Once the 40 seconds has expired, return to your base level for 60 seconds. Observe your heart rate reaching to the mid-70% of maximum BPM during the 40-second sprint.

In the second move, increase incline/resistance a step and once again accelerate cadence in a burst to the 110+ range for 40 seconds. Observe your heart rate BPM ticking up to the upper 70% range of maximum BPM. At the end of the 40-second burst, reduce cadence and incline/resistance, returning to your base level for 60 seconds before executing the third move.

In the third and final move, increase incline/resistance a step above the last move (to 12) and again, in a burst of acceleration, increase cadence to the 110+ RPM level for 40 seconds. Observe your heart rate BPM reaching 80% of maximum BPM. At the end of the segment, execute a 1-minute recovery.

Starting Out of the Saddle–This is a slightly more intense form of sprints. Like the preceding in the saddle version, this form of sprint also executes three moves but is different by simply starting each move by coming out of the saddle for 5 seconds while accelerating toward 110+ RPM, and then returning to the saddle for the remainder of the 40-second sprint.

As with the in the saddle sprint, the first move starts by increasing incline/resistance from your base; however, since you will be coming out of the saddle, you will increase incline/resistance to 11 and come out of the saddle while increasing your cadence in a burst of acceleration for a 5 count, before returning to the saddle to maintain 110 RPM for the remainder of the 40 seconds.

Once the 40 seconds has expired, return to your base level for 60 seconds. Observe your heart rate reaching to the mid-70% of maximum BPM. Repeat the second and third moves in similar fashion, increasing incline/resistance a step to start each as you come out of the saddle for a 5 count and quickly accelerate RPM to the 110 RPM level, and maintaining this cadence for the remainder of each 40-second move. Observe your heart rate BPM increase to the 80–83% of maximum BPM in these moves. At the end of the segment, execute a 1-minute recovery.

Varying Incline/Resistance, Duration, and Cadence–Use caution as you work sprints into your spin session. Particularly when using the starting out of the saddle version, it is necessary for you to be comfortable with the incline/resistance, durations, and cadence illustrated above. Always make it YOUR RIDE.

For some, the 40-second sprint duration will be too much; so, make it 20 or 30 seconds and adjust the base time. Same with incline/resistance step-ups. Make them something you can do and repeat each time you spin. Same thing for those who are able to sprint longer at higher levels of incline/resistance. Again, make it YOUR RIDE.

In any event, sprints can be very exhausting, so at the end of your sprint segment, execute a 1-minute recovery.

Running Jumps (4 minutes)

As was the case with the basic jumps described in Chapter 3, running jumps are performed simply by coming out of the saddle from your base for an 8 count, to either a standing position or an out extended position with your butt raised just above the saddle. Your hands are either where they were in the base position if standing, or extended. Incline/resistance is easy to moderate.

The running jump move differs in that as you leave the saddle, you accelerate cadence to 90+ RPM for an 8 count before returning to the seated base position for 8 seconds before jumping and accelerating out of the saddle again, running for another 8 seconds before returning to base. The running jumps are repeated for the duration of the segment (e.g., 4 minutes) and typically heart rate will reach the 72–79% of maximum BPM during the run, as opposed to 70% of maximum BPM with basic jumps. At the end of the running jumps segment, execute a 1-minute recovery.

I often use a segment of running jumps near the end of my spin session as a means of keeping my heart rate elevated longer before the cooldown or at the start of the challenge portion of my session to elevate my heart rate earlier in the ride.

Be careful to monitor the impact of this move on your knees and make adjustments to the number of jumps, segment duration, incline/resistance, etc., if you discover soreness, tightness, or any discomfort, especially later in the day or the following day. Consider using another move in place of jumps if the move bothers your knees.

CHAPTER 5 SUMMARY

In this chapter, the Structured Spinning session is expanded upon with the presentation of a structured 60-minute spin session, illustrated in chart form, that is used by the author. The reader is informed of the availability of a blank chart (i.e., a spin session design aid) by emailing Structured_Spinning@Yahoo.com. Also, the additional moves used in the 60-minute session are explained: running jumps, standing incline, seated incline, and sprints.

CHAPTER 6

Closing Notes

As this guide comes to a close, I want to leave you with a few final thoughts to keep in mind as you spin forward in your health and fitness journey.

PREP FOR THE WORLD SERIES

Think of your Structured Spinning sessions like the baseball season. Over the course of the baseball season, it's not the outcome of any single game that matters. Rather, it's what is learned from each game that enables each player and the team to improve over the course of the season to be the best they can be by the end of the season and make it to the World Series.

So too with spinning. This is where the distinction I make comes in with regard to variable spin class sessions at a club versus the Structured Spinning solo method with its measured continuity and repeatability in supporting planned improvement and longevity. Earlier I talked about the lack of continuity from one health club class to the next. Here's an example:

> Ms. Smith leads spin class on Tuesday, John Doe on Thursday, and Billy Bob on Saturday. Spinning in each of these three instructor's classes often results in Ms. Smith hitting the mark, and you come away feeling like you had a good workout and enjoyed the music. She provided some structure to the session by targeting heart rate, using cadence, incline, and duration targets, etc. Then, on Tuesday, just when you're excited and hoping to build on the previous class, John Doe has the lights off so you can't read your heart rate

monitor or the bike's display, and there's no structure to the session because he has a hangover and is taking it easy by just going through the motions. You come away from the session thinking you just wasted 45 minutes. Then, on Saturday, the young stud instructor, Billy Bob, ramps up the session, and you're exhausted after the first 18 minutes . . . another disappointment. I'm sure we've all been through this or a similar sequence of disappointing sessions; and, if not, just wait, it's coming.

You see, in any event, this day-to-day approach misses the point of Structured Spinning—i.e., it's not about any one, two, or three sessions; it's about a lifetime of fitness improvement and overall health maintenance. It's about the next 20, 30, or more sessions and how you improve, reinforce, and/or maintain your conditioning based on your current level of fitness and energy. What is important about each session is what you learn about your level of fitness and how/where to improve from one session to the next and, over time, building on the previous session(s) so that there is an unbroken and consistent operation over the season of life.

Think of how professional baseball teams train during the 162-game season played over approximately six months. In each game, win or lose, what is important is what the manager, coaches, and players learn in order to improve and make changes so that, the next time they play, they are a better team that enables them to win.

Structured Spinning enables a similar approach through your observation of the measures discussed in the methodology to build a chain of improvement from session to session, and by adjusting a repeatable workout structure if and where necessary by, for example, adding/modifying segments to target a higher BPM heart rate or targeting a higher calorie burn at the end of the next session, accomplishing a higher level of work by increasing time and cadence over a defined period of time.

So, it's not any one, two, or three session, but how you are performing your sessions over an extended period of weeks and months and whether you are building strength and/or maintaining your level of fitness as measured by the indications I've set out in Structured Spinning.

Under normal circumstances, that will be the case; *inevitably*, however, *there will be* injuries, illness, multiweek layoffs due to vacations, etc. When you can return to your regular workout session, the first day/week back may be a struggle to execute your "usual" session; in this case, you need to identify where you are off and make a plan by adjusting your spin session in order to safely get back to where you were before your layoff. Maybe your heart rate is less than the BPM targets you're used to hitting and/or your quads are burning and tired during the seated incline segment, etc.

The question now is, "How can I get back to where I was before vacation, illness, etc.?" With Structured Spinning, you can set a course back to where you were by starting with easier sessions, which you design yourself, and slowly increase intensity over several sessions before reaching the level you were at before the layoff. Then, from there, you may target a higher intensity of spinning or perhaps just maintain the fitness level you're at. Regardless, you will overcome the weakness(es) brought on by the layoff and come back a winner, feeling like you've made it to the World Series!

MOTIVATION

When I've discussed spinning and the Structured Spinning methodology, I'm occasionally asked about motivation. During my first couple years in spin class, I remember feeling motivated by trying to perform at the level of others in the class and/or by following the instructor's commands. Many people have told me that they are motivated by being in this environment. Likewise, internet-connected spin bikes create a similar setting.

So where do you find motivation spinning solo at home or in an empty spin studio? The answer is through self-motivation by challenging yourself to reach the targets you set out for yourself. Granted, self-motivation may not work for everyone, and for some, the class setting delivers a social lift regardless of the workout. But what I discovered after using the Structured Spinning method for a while is that I was self-motivating myself just as much and more than the instructor du jour, and I enjoyed challenging myself with additional segments, higher heart rate targets, extending durations as I ran up the hill, and simply by personally designing my sessions. So, guess what? In the end, you'll surprise yourself at how motivated you are to be as good as you can be. All you needed were the tools that Structured Spinning gives you.

DESIGN YOUR OWN SPIN MOVES

Needless to say, there are several spinning moves besides the ones I've included in this guide. Just to mention a couple that are popular are those where you raise your butt slightly off the saddle with hands/arms extended out and those that target strengthening the upper body by raising and lowering the chest to and from the handlebars as if doing pushups. The former butt-raising form is often performed with sprints, jumps, or any other move where you come out of the saddle for a period.

These are good examples of how you can adapt moves to target muscle groups. In the first case, the glutes, hamstring, quads, and back muscles are targeted in this advanced move. The latter, which is a low-level intensity move and can be executed as part of several of the moves discussed, strengthens the upper-body muscles, including the arms, chest, and shoulder.

On occasion I've also seen people spinning with light weights in their hands and using these in arm-strengthening moves while in the saddle and spinning.

So, take note and be creative with care. Experiment and try to develop new moves and adapt your existing ones by watching for ideas from the greater cycling world—indoors, outdoors, and virtually.

INCLINE/RESISTANCE AND OTHER SPIN BIKE SETTINGS

Throughout this guide I've suggested incline/resistance and other spin bike settings. It should be clearly understood that particularly with incline/resistance, spin bike settings can be significantly different from one bike to another, even when the bikes in a spin studio are the same make and model. The difference is typically minor, but sometimes it can be significant, especially when moving between health clubs where the bike is something other than what you're used to. This is especially true if you expect to spin while traveling. In these instances, it is necessary for you, the rider, to check and modify the settings in preparation for your ride to ensure safety, comfort, and a productive ride.

So, if you're not spinning at home on your own bike and using those in your local health club, find a bike, or better yet, a few bikes in the studio where you spin, and use those particular ones as often as possible. This is not a hard thing to do since most clubs have identifying numbers on each of their bikes for inventory, manufacturer warranty, and/or maintenance identification.

SEGMENT LENGTH

You may be wondering why Structure Spinning segments are 4 minutes. In general, they're just right with the 1-minute recovery to make up a total 5-minute segment. So, it's just a timing thing for me and should not stop you from designing *your* moves and segments to suit *your* needs. If a 12-minute seated incline segment is your cup of tea . . . go for it! Make it YOUR RIDE!

CHAPTER 6 SUMMARY

In this chapter, the author adds a few final thoughts about spinning in general and the Structured Spinning methodology in this guide. He presents an interesting analogy between Structured Spinning and how a pro baseball team learns its strengths and weakness from each game and makes adjustments during the season in order to be on top at the end of the season—so too with spinning. Each session is planned, measured, and adjustments made going forward to reach your health goals over the long haul. He points out how the structured spin method requires self-motivation and how this can be achieved despite spinning "solo." Creativity in designing your own self-fulfilling moves is emphasized as well as key points about moving between spin bikes and how their settings and readings can differ significantly. Finally, the author points out that the 4-minute segments used in the guide are merely what he likes to use, and it should not discourage the reader from designing shorter or longer segments.

SS Session Design Aid

Segment	Move	Hands/ Position	Duration	Incline/ Resistance	Cadence/ RPM	Heart Rate/ BPM
1						
2						
3						
4						
5						
6						
7						
8						
9						
10						
11						

Segment	Move	Hands/ Position	Duration	Incline/ Resistance	Cadence/ RPM	Heart Rate/ BPM
12						
13						
14						
15						
16						
17						
18						
19						
20						
21						
22						
23						
24						
25						

Request a PDF of this chart to download and print
by emailing Structured_Spinning@Yahoo.com.

Index

Page numbers in italics refer to photographs.

About the Author

Joel Malek is a retired information technology consultant who has authored works of both fiction and nonfiction. Of Polish descent, he was born in Greenpoint, Brooklyn, New York, and grew up on Eastern Long Island during the late fifties, playing Little League baseball, touch football, and hockey in the shadows of the Long Island Arena.

In his early teens, he learned to ski and was fortunate to have family living in Ludlow, Vermont, with a very accommodative weekend visit policy.

He graduated from SUNY at Stony Brook in New York, earning a BA, and later an MBA from Manhattan College in Riverdale, Bronx, New York. In 1976, he married his wife, Patricia. They lived for several years in Middle Village, Queens, New York, where Joel began playing paddle ball and competitive racquetball.

During his career as an information technology consultant, he worked at the "C" level with upper management at Credit Suisse, Sony Music, Con Agra, Prime Computer, and several others, integrating enterprise-wide business solutions across numerous IT platforms.

When not traveling, the Maleks reside in the town of Port Washington, New York, located along the Gold Coast of Long Island's North Shore. Now retired, the author spends his time doing research for upcoming works, writing, playing guitar, golfing, skiing, and spinning of course.

CPSIA information can be obtained
at www.ICGtesting.com
Printed in the USA
BVHW051500141121
621552BV00005B/52